(Not Just)

Your Everyday Stretch Book

Written by Austin Stack
with Illustrations by Ariel Ciprian

Order this book online at www.trafford.com
or email orders@trafford.com

Most Trafford titles are also available at major online book retailers.

Printed in Victoria, BC, Canada.

ISBN: 978-1-4269-3413-1 (sc)

*Our mission is to efficiently provide the world's finest, most comprehensive book publishing
service, enabling every author to experience success. To find out how to publish your book, your
way, and have it available worldwide, visit us online at www.trafford.com*

Trafford rev. 5/20/2010

Trafford
PUBLISHING®   www.trafford.com

North America & international
toll-free: 1 888 232 4444 (USA & Canada)
phone: 250 383 6864 ♦ fax: 812 355 4082

INTRODUCTION

Blessed are those who run around in circles for they shall be known as wheels...

This proverb is one of the first clues I had as an adult as to what I was like as a child. I had some distilled memories from childhood but I am not one of those people that can remember what my life was like or what I was like as a child from an early age. Some people claim that they remember events from as early 1 or 2 years old. That would definitely not be me. My memories are more scattered as I mostly recall highlights. But I have held onto to a transition item from my childhood given to me by my mother. It was a little metal tray with the above written proverb on it. I never gave it much thought when I was growing up but realized in adulthood that this was a kind of message from my Mom or so I would like to think. The message, I suppose, is that this is how my mother perceived me as a child. So it gives me a glimpse into what I must have been like growing up. Did I really run around in circles? I guess it's possible but I believe it refers more to my need as a child, as much as my need as an adult, to move. To constantly be in motion.

I have always been active as both a child and an adult although I never really participated in organized sports partly from a lack of any real competitive spirit. I have never felt the need to compete with other people. I lack the competitive gene. But I do have a need for movement. I have always loved swimming, biking, walking, hiking, dancing, and I slowly introduced new activities as I entered adulthood. As an adult, weight training has endured as my primary physical activity. I have been weight training for 27 years. I actually started fooling around in a gym when I was in college. For many years, it was just a part time hobby. I soon became more serious about weight training upon my arrival in San Francisco, and started to regularly use the campus gymnasium as a way to fend off any and all stress while attending San Francisco State. I soon found that I could center myself emotionally through the sets and repetitions like a mantra of sorts. I consider weight training to be an active form of meditation. It suited me both emotionally and physically. There is (was) no competition except with myself. The counting of repetitions and the physical movement of the weights was soothing. I was, of course, also very skinny and noticed that my body was changing as a result of the weight training. I had always wanted to be bigger and stronger, and admired all of the old classic bodybuilders of the day. Again, I wanted this for myself.

I had no need to prove anything to anyone else. That was in 1982 when I was 26 years old. I am now 53 years old.

This book is a result of my years of weight training and, of course, stretching. I spent the next several years of my early adulthood reading everything I could about the sport. I do not like to think of my sport as bodybuilding but I suppose this is probably as a good a description as any other way to describe what I engage in on an almost daily basis. Bodybuilding has a lot of negative connotations for me related to ego and narcissism. I prefer the term of weight training. I essentially self-educated myself about the most efficient and effective way to achieve the results I wanted for my body. My desire was to become more muscular and stronger than I had been as a child, and I wanted to do it as smartly as I could in the shortest amount of time. It is my nature as a New Yorker to get in and get out of the gym as quickly as possible. I still have the same perspective. I could go into all of the routines I have learned after years of reading and actual weight training but you could simply pick up one of the many bodybuilding books that are out there and read for yourself. There are some basic rules of weight training that have been around since the early days, and there has not been much change to these core principles. I am not interested in rewriting what has already been said a million times but please know that concepts like muscle confusion have been around for a long time. You can buy any standard bodybuilding book, and learn these principles as well.

I always have an eye toward effectiveness and efficiency. Many people at the gym waste a lot of time and effort because they do not know what they are doing, even those with trainers because not all trainers are equal. I am not into all these fad systems or exercise programs of the month. Nothing is better than consistency, training with weights, and mental focus. Other tricks such as always start with the big muscles and move toward the smaller muscles both within an individual workout and your overall weekly routine.

This book is about stretching, though. And primarily about stretching because I believe that I have, over the years, constructed a unique approach to warming up. My system of stretching is one that you can use and carry with you through your life… maybe even add years of vitality and health. It's smart, simple, and comprehensive. Other stretching books are not going to provide you with as an efficient and effective routine. Stretching is crucial to successful participation in a sport. It does not matter what sport although this is probably best suited to weight training. This book is also best for those individuals who have some sports background, and stretching experience already in their repertoire. I will demonstrate how to complete the stretches in the particular sequence that I have developed so as to finish quickly and efficiently. Again, no waste of time or energy. You need that energy to devote to the sport or, in my case, the lifting of weights.

For me, stretching is not a sport in and of itself. It is a prelude and a conclusion to my sport of weight training. Having said that, I believe that for some people that stretching alone or in combination with yoga maybe the best form of physical exercise for them. But for those who are involved in a sport, it is then important to conserve your primary energy toward that sport, and less energy toward the warm-up. Stretching is just that, a warm up and should not take more then 30 minutes. Too much time spent in stretching can take away the energy needed to lift weights or engage in your sport.

But it is important to warm up your muscles before engaging in any athletic activity. Stretching increases the blood flow, and literally warms up the muscles in preparation of exercising. If your muscles are "cold" and you engage in a sport or physical activity then you are likely to experience an injury. You should only read this book if you have come to your sport especially if it's weight training with the attitude that I'm here, first and foremost, for my health. Because that is really what this is all about. Most importantly, stretching will contribute greatly to your overall health, and ability to participate in your sport without injury. I have been working out for 27 years, and I can count on two hands the number of times I have had an injury. If you are experiencing injuries then this book is for you. Stretching is for you. Weight training or any other sport with repetitive movement requires that you stretch. The repetitive movement adds additional stress over and above the normal wear and tear that your body goes through as it ages. Much like carpel tunnel syndrome you can experience similar pain and joint problems. Stretching has inherent health benefits for your body outside of the single focus of a sport or as an adjunct to a sport. A lot of the stretching I do comes directly from runners but also from people who practice yoga. Yoga has a whole mind-body connection that will prepare for your sport as well as for life. Stretching will make you a better athlete and maybe a better person. It will help to center you emotionally, and increase your ability to focus on your sport. If you are bodybuilding then you must make the mind-body connection in order to fully reap the benefits from lifting weights. If all you are doing is swinging weights around without "feeling" the muscles doing the work then you will never fully realize your potential. You need to focus and feel the specific muscle group making the effort. For example, when you are doing back exercises you need to make sure that the back muscles are meeting the resistance, and not your arms or shoulders. If you engage in stretching especially stretching from a mind-body perspective then you can learn how to isolate the "feel" of the individual muscle groups. This ability to have a complete sense of your body (muscles) in action as in yoga, in turn, can be used when you are actually working out those muscle groups.

I think most of us see the body as immutable. I know that, in fact, you can change your body through sports/weight training. I have been able to change my body from being incredibly skinny (125 lbs) to bigger and more muscular (155 lbs). It has taken a very long time for me to achieve these results without the use of any drugs. There are no healthy shortcuts. If you want faster results then I suggest you find alternative methods because this book is not for you. This is not a fad…it takes hard work and time to change your body and to achieve a balance of the physical and mental elements in your life. There are no short cuts. The stretches I use during this 30 minute routine are not especially unique unto themselves. The secret to my stretches lies in the sequencing. They should be done before you work out (or engage in a sport) and then, afterwards whereby you can do a modified/shortened version or similar cool down activity.

This set of stretches will cover the entire musculature of the body in a methodical manner whereby there is no loss of energy or effort. It follows a set routine to be copied by the reader with narrative and pictures. There are no shortcuts. Some stretches may not be achievable immediately but can be carried out to the best of the reader's ability and modified as to their current and on-going flexibility. Some days may prove easier than others or it may simply take time to achieve the full range of the stretch. Be patient, and enjoy feeling stronger and more flexible overtime.

The stretches described in this book are primarily directed toward those with some history of stretching already but may also be used by individuals new to stretching. Stretching is inherently critical to any sport but especially those sports with repetitive movements such as weight training. Adding a program of yoga to the series would prove beneficial. These stretches are to be done on days that you engage in your sport. The stretches have been pre-determined to cover all muscle groups, and are to be done in the order as noted in the book. Following this predetermined order contributes to the overall effectiveness, and efficiency of the stretching. Some variation is allowed, of course, but it is suggested to keep the stretching to no more than 30 minutes. You do not want to stress or pre-fatigue the muscles as conservation of effort is critical. Although the focus is upon pre-exercise stretching or warming up; it is equally important to cool down. The cool down stretches may be shorter in length, and may not necessarily follow the predetermined routine.

Stretches are done carefully, slowly, and should never hurt. Remember to breathe. You want to increase the range of motion over time. Just as in weight training, you want to achieve a full range of motion when stretching. For example, reaching for your toes may be very difficult for you. You may have to start with resting your hand on your ankle instead. If you feel pain while engaged in a stretch then stop immediately. Absolutely no bouncing! You will increase your range of flexibility through consistent and deliberate effort. Pressure overtime.

You do not need to be in a gym in order to follow this stretching routine. You will need a flat surface, a mat if you like, and a pole. As a weight trainer I am interested in sculpting my body. Stretching can also afford an opportunity to accomplish this endeavor as well. So there are some stretches that are geared specifically toward the waistline with the added benefit of reducing your waistline while preparing to engage in a sport. This stretching routine does necessarily address your "core" better known as your midsection but there is some potential benefit to your waistline. The purpose here is to reduce not enlarge your midsection. Here are some tips related to your waistline. When doing abdominal exercises use your own bodyweight or light weights otherwise you will increase your overall girth. Use little to no weights when doing sit-ups or side bends. The illustration precedes the written description so that you, the reader, can see the movement.

Focus and feel the stretch!

***<u>WARNING: DO THESE STRETCHES ONLY WITH
AND UNDER THE ADVICE OF A PHYSICIAN!</u>***

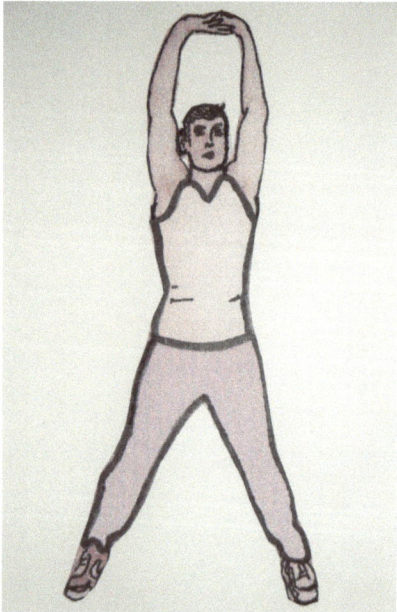
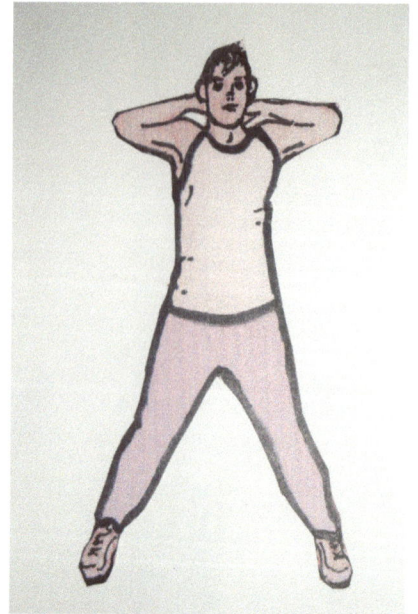
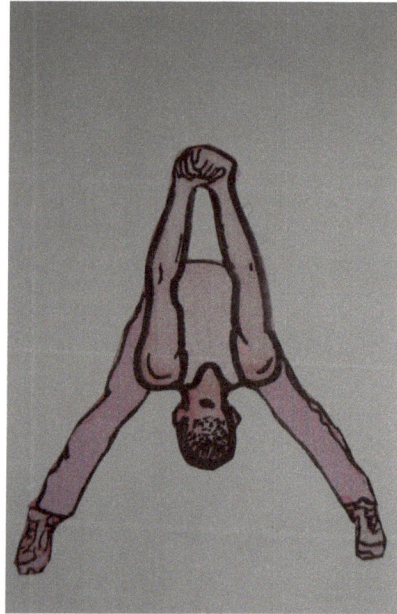
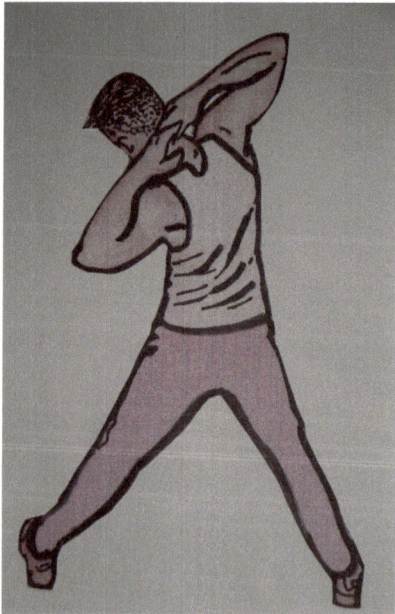
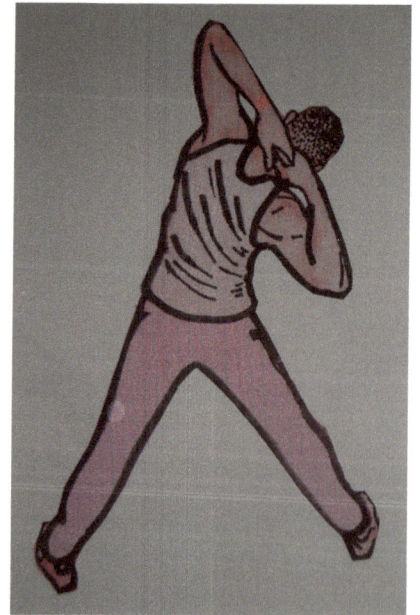

Stand, and Reach I (2 minutes max)
(stance: slightly wider than hip distance apart)

This first stretch is just that. A chance to stretch out your body. Stand with your feet slightly wider than hip distant apart. Clasp hands in front of your body by intertwining fingers and turn the clasp inside out as you reach for the sky. Then as you lower your arms, release the clasp, grab one hand in the other and pull as you move your arms behind your head. Then twist your upper body to the each side. Left and right. Let go of the clasp. Lower your arms and then grab one hand with the other behind your back, and lift your arms up over your head, bend forward while at the same time bending your knees slightly. Hang in that position for a few seconds with your pinkies over your head and facing the ground. While hanging in that position you can (very carefully) straighten your legs while leaving only a slight bend in the knees. Focus and feel the stretch!

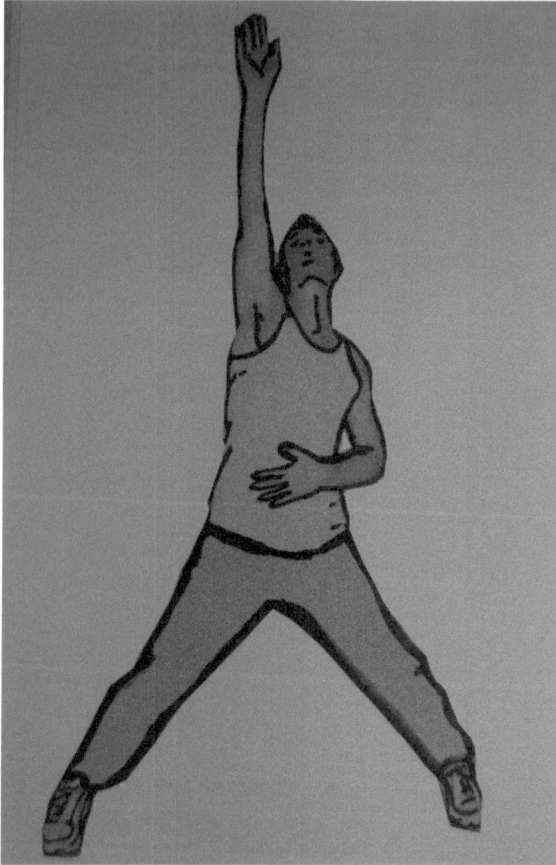
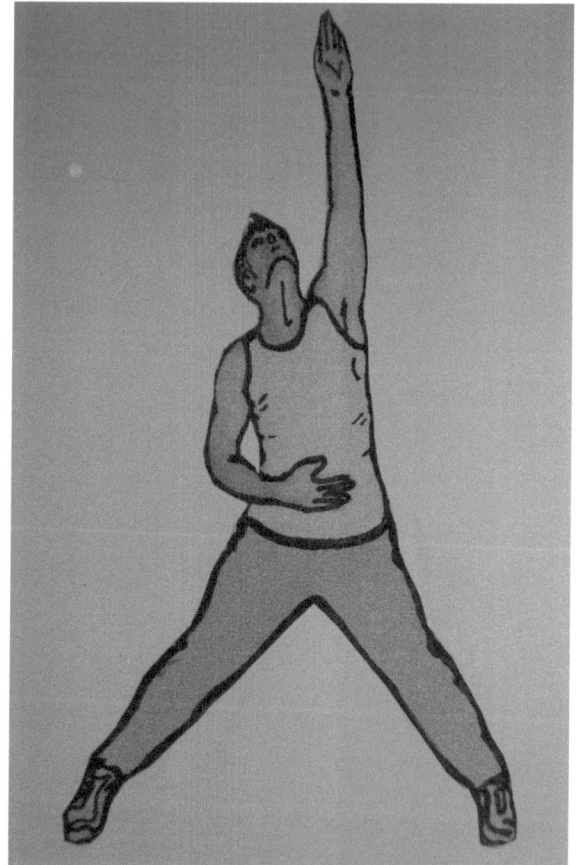

Stand and Reach II (2 minutes max) (stance: slightly wider than hip distance apart)

Raise both arms in the air from your sides in a sweeping motion. Alternately reach upwards with both arms (palms facing toward each other) much like the in the yoga position known as the *raised hands pose*. Then release both arms down alongside your body. Now, alternately reach with both arms (palms facing forward)…getting a maximum stretch on each side by trying to extend a little further each time. You can do this by alternating arms several times. For a slightly different stretch, turns palms outward and/or raise both arms simultaneously. Focus and feel the stretch!

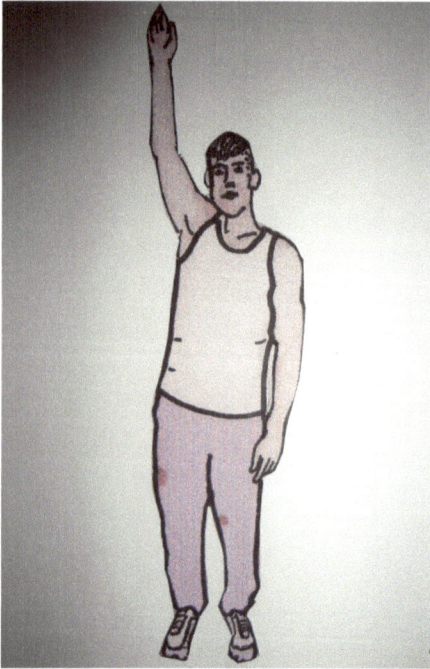
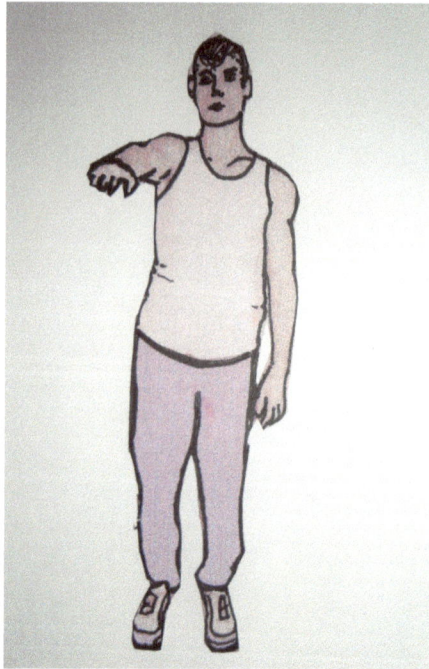
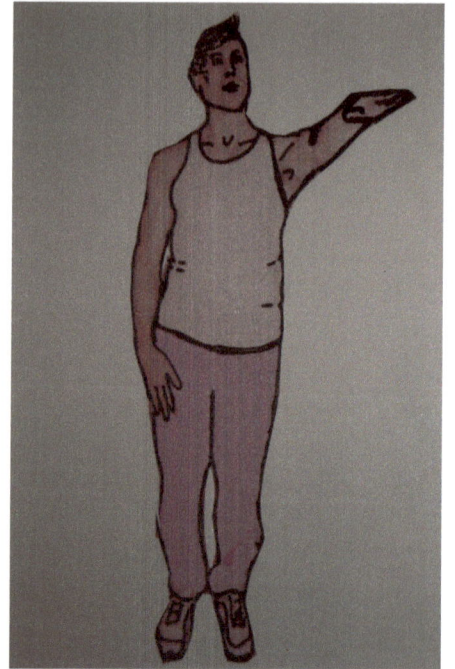
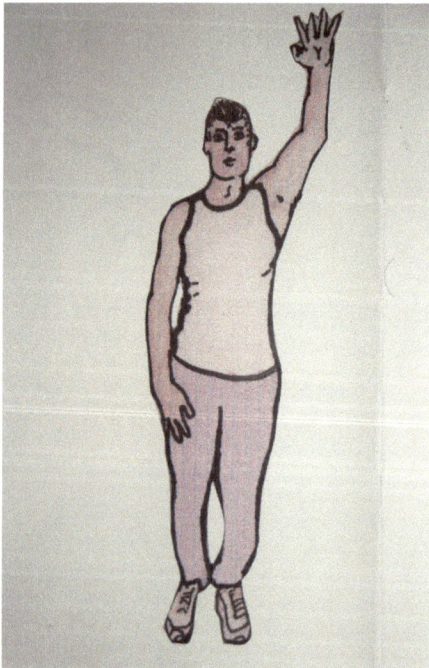
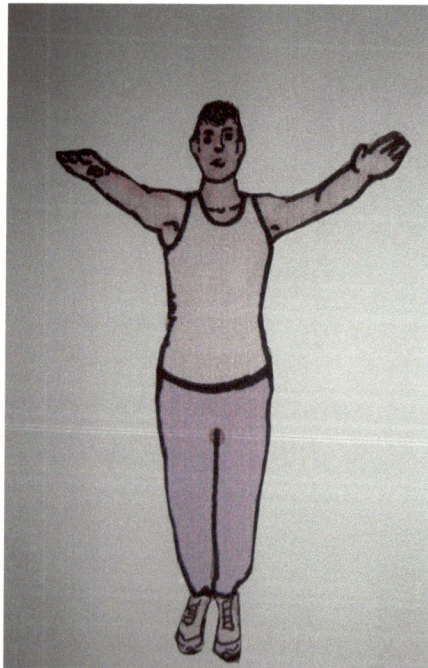
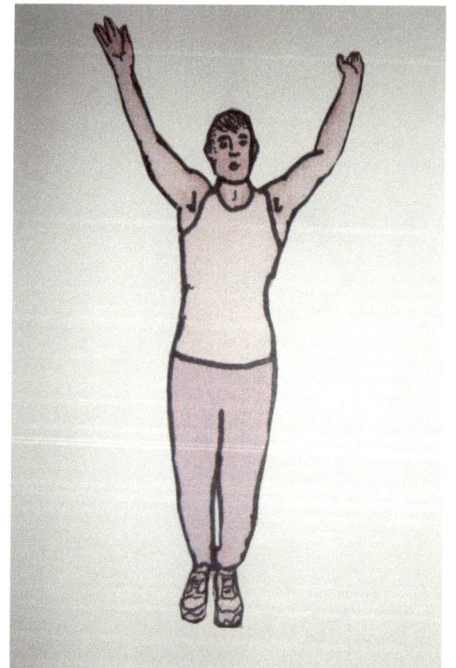

12

Arm Swings (2 minutes max) (feet hip distant apart)

Start swinging your arms while crossing your midline. Then baseball swings of each individual arm forward and then backward. Then both arms at the same time forward and backward simultaneously. Focus and feel the stretch!

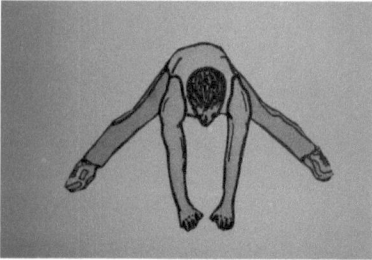
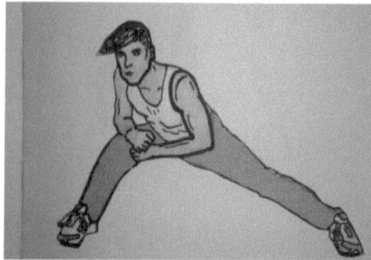
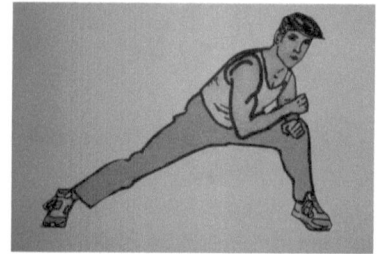

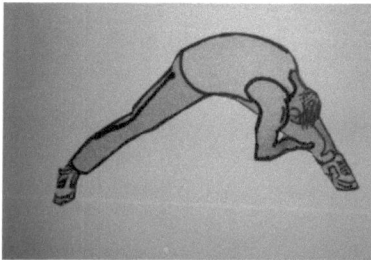
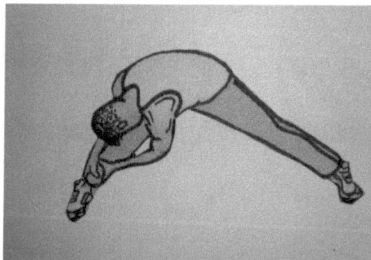
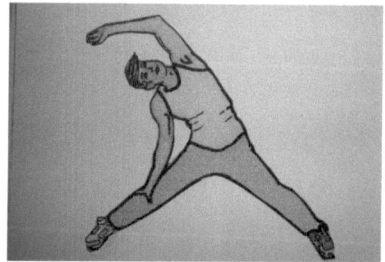

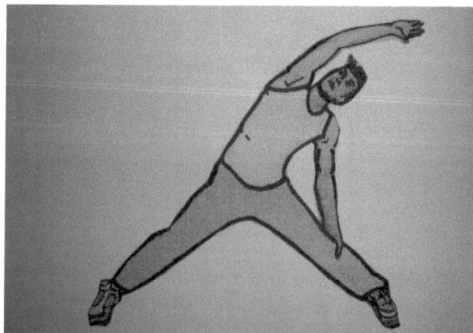

14

Leg stretch (2 minutes max) (wide leg stance)

Stretch your legs out wide as wide as you can go without bending your knees. Lean into and down so that your upper torso is hanging from your hips. Neck and head relaxed. Hang for a moment. Your back is flat at first then you can lower into the stretch. Place both hands on your ankles. Next, move both hands to one ankle and then both hands to the other ankle while pulling your torso into your knees. Now raise your torso upright and lean with an outstretched arm toward the opposite side of your body. Try to lean into the stretch so that your torso is facing front and hips are reaching toward the sky. Do the same movement on the other side. Focus and feel the stretch!

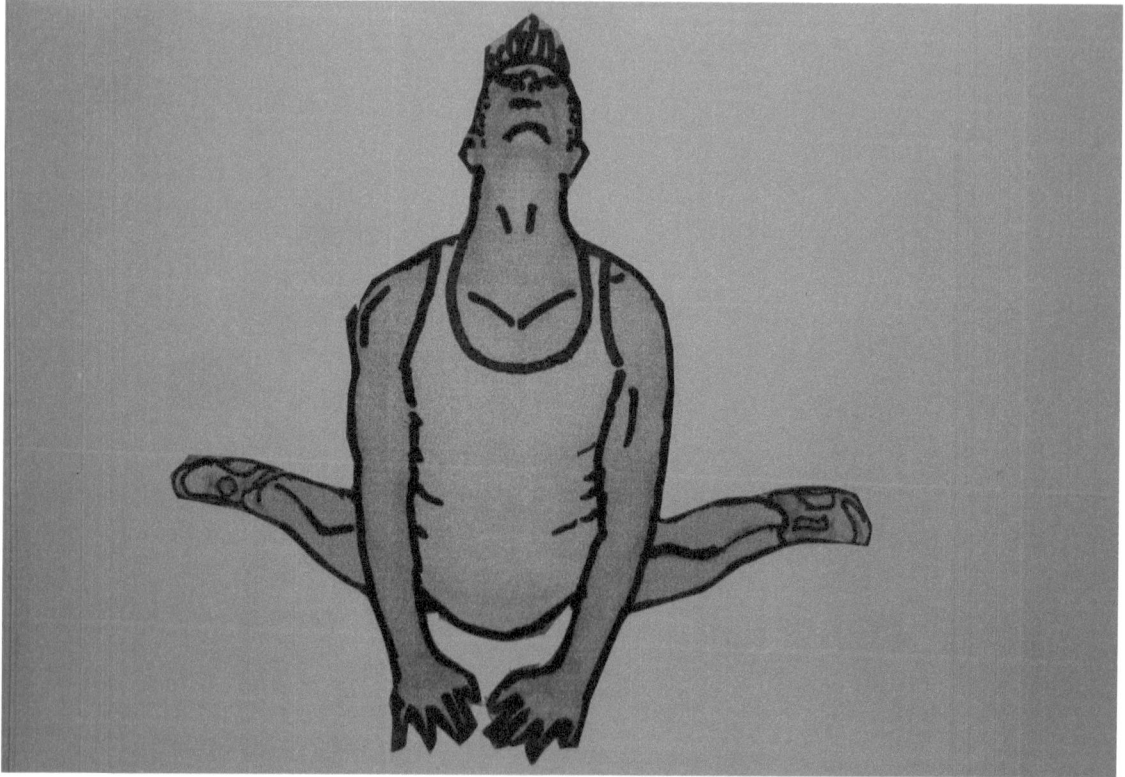

Upward Dog I (2 minutes max) (wide leg stance)

With your legs remaining in the same wide stance bring your body forward using your arms while leaving the legs in the same position as your arms reach out and lower your body to the floor. Your arms are now supporting your upper torso and you are stretching upward with shoulders down and chest up. You can lean toward each side to feel the stretch in your obliques. You should feel this stretch in both the front and back of your upper body as well as in your legs. Your legs are resting on the mat and your upper body is raised off the floor with the support and strength of your arms. Focus and feel the stretch!

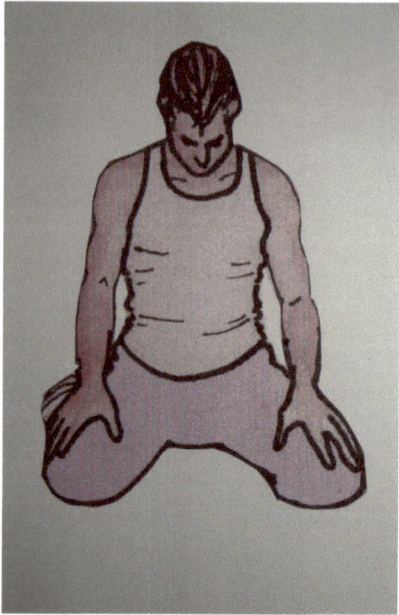
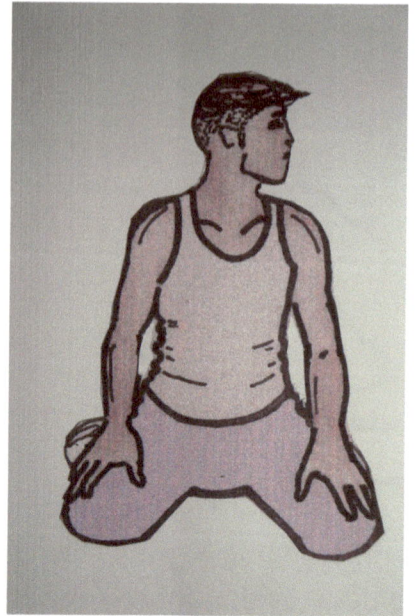
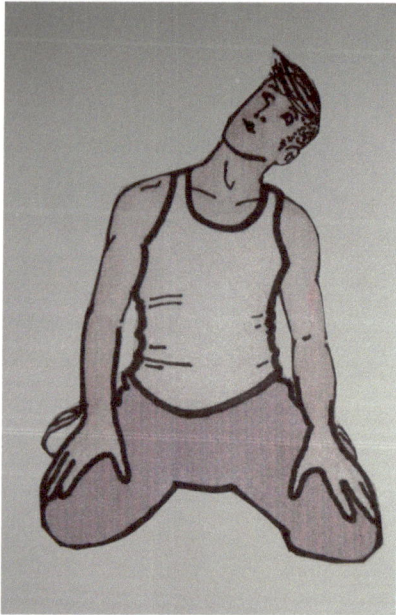
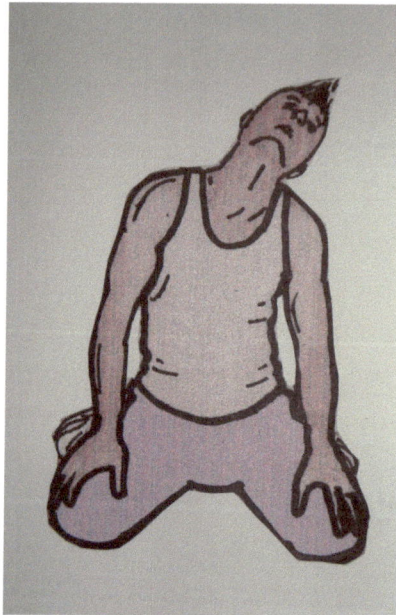
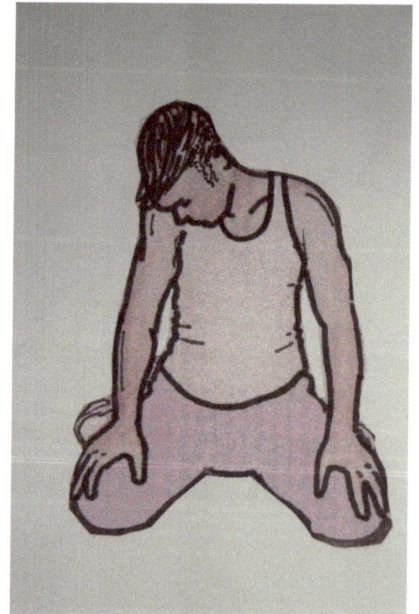

Neck Stretch (2 minutes max)

Now, simply lean back from the previous position and sit down on the mat. You can sit in any position that is comfortable. I usually sit in a frog like position with my feet facing the back wall. While in this sitting position I loosen up my neck muscles with a series of carefully controlled, slow movements. First, nod your head backward and forward. Then roll your head from side to side. Then turn your head from side to side. Now, roll your head in semi circles leading into full circles. Never roll your head in semi or full circles without warming up the neck first. Focus and feel the stretch!

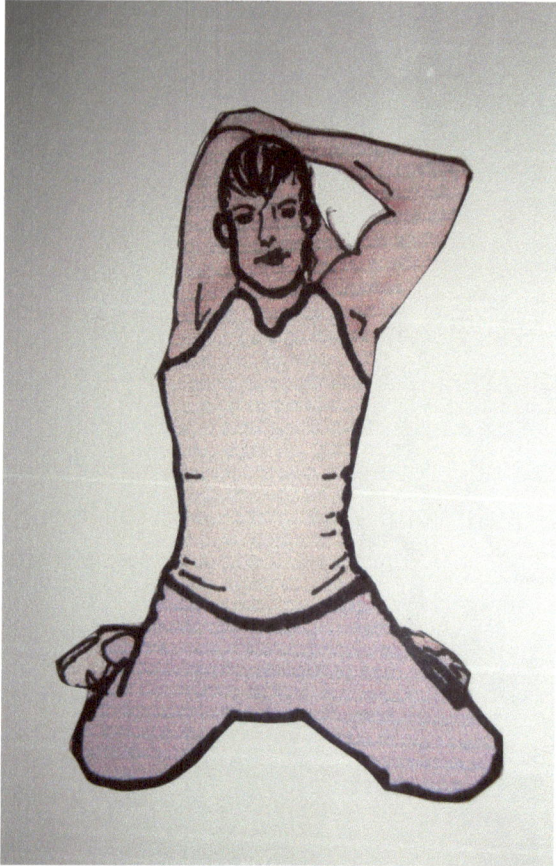

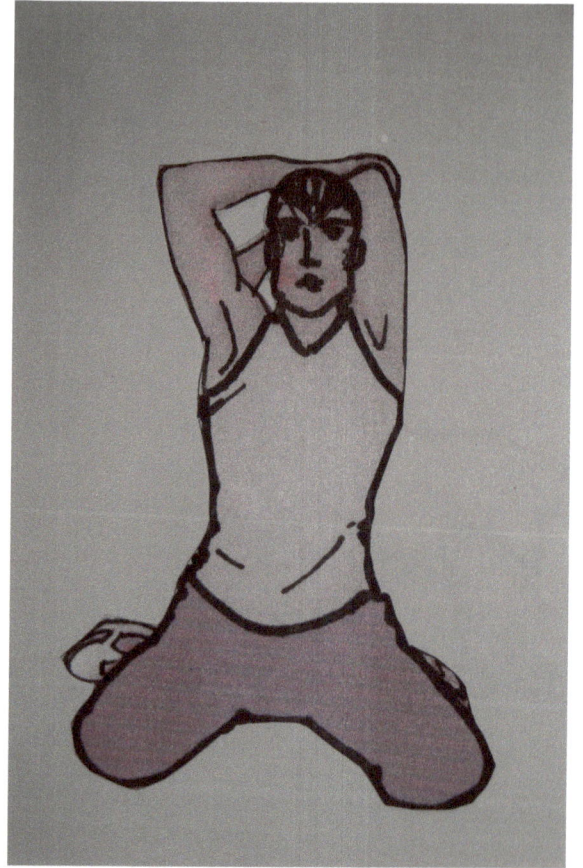

Triceps Stretch (2 minutes max)

I also take time to stretch out the triceps, shoulders and back again by raising one arm over your head, grabbing your elbow with the opposite hand and pulling gently then complete on opposite side. Keep your head and neck relaxed but erect. Focus and feel the stretch!

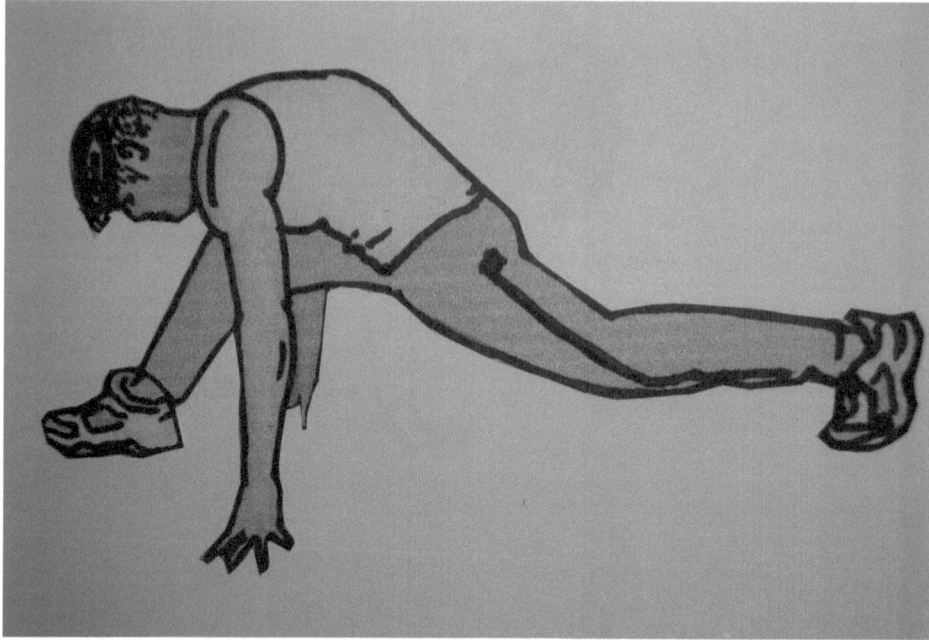
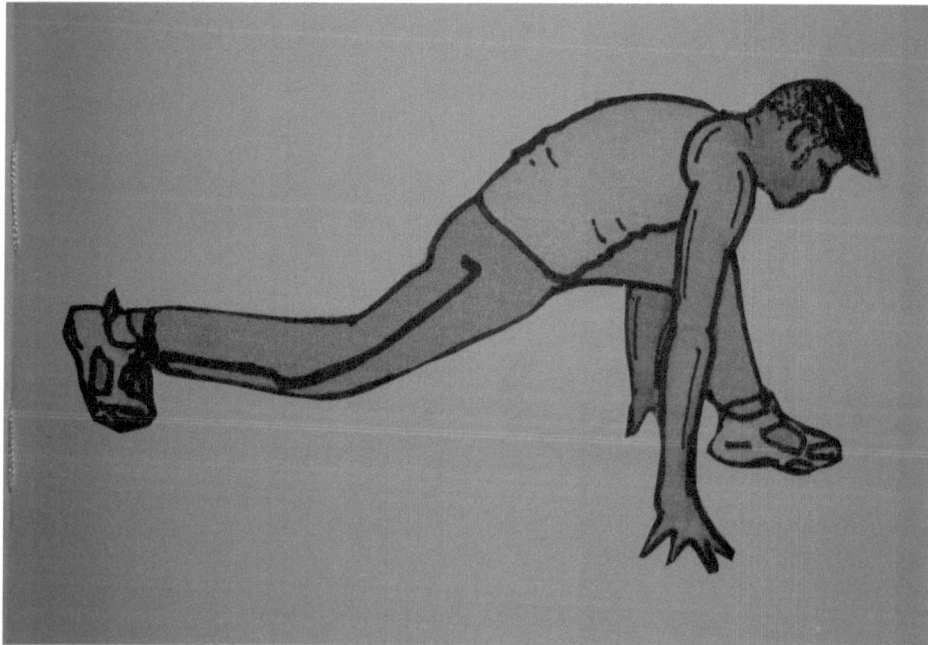

Leg stretches (2 minutes max) (wide leg)

Now, return to the original standing position with a wide leg stance and while turning it parallel to the front wall. Then change the position of your upper torso and legs by turning sideways and toward the left (or right), bending the front knee (90 degree angle), placing your hands on both sides of the front knee and stretching the back leg back while keeping it straight with the knee off of the ground. Your front knee is bent at a 90 degree angle and the back knee does not touch the ground. You can play with the position of your back foot by turning it in, under or to the side while remaining in the same position. Turn and face the other direction using the same knee and foot positions. Focus and feel the stretch!

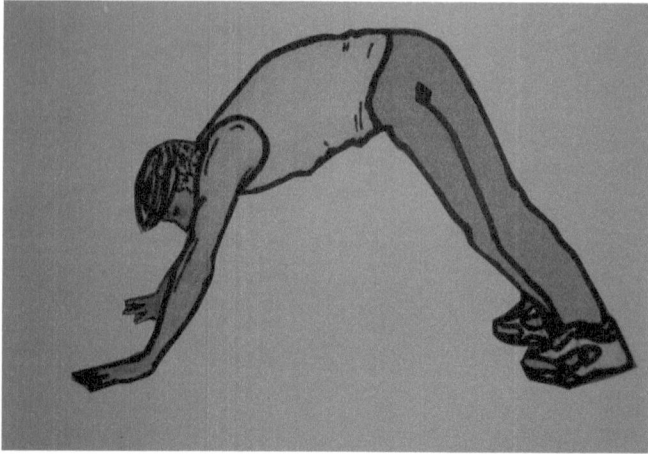
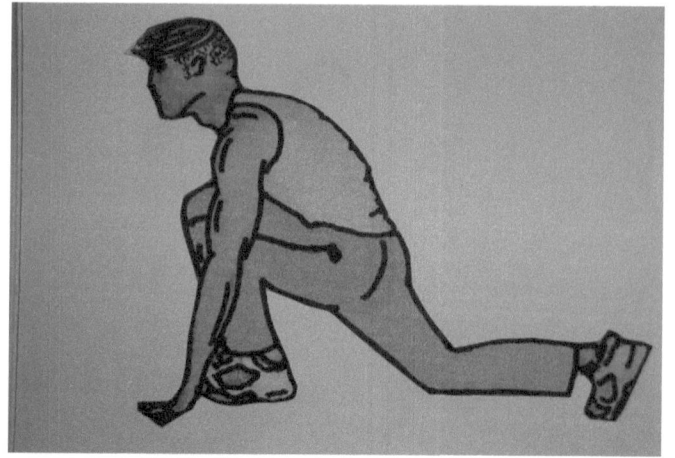
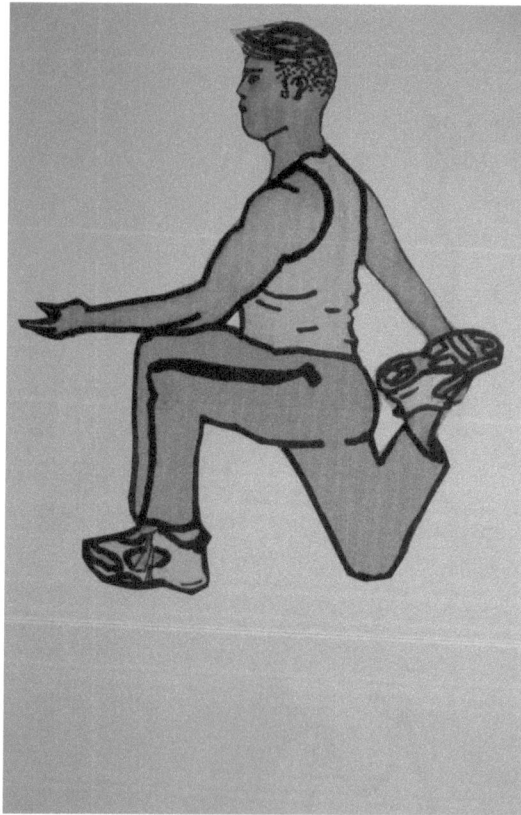

Downward Facing Dog & Leg Stretch (2 minutes max) (feet hip distance apart)

From the previous stretch, bring your front leg back and move into a downward dog. Move the mat back and closer toward your feet so your arms are in front and your legs are behind the mat. Raise one leg at a time while remaining in downward facing dog.

Bring the right (or left) leg out and back away from your body then as you bring it back towards you, move it into position between your hands. Your front knee is bent at a 90 degree angle with hands on each side of your front knee while bringing down the back knee to rest on the mat. Raise your torso (sit up) using your arms and rest your elbow onto your knee (right elbow on front right knee or left elbow on left front knee). Bend your back leg and with the opposite hand grab that ankle and pull toward your body. Use this hand to hold onto your raised back leg and foot. For a deeper stretch, raise your torso into a higher position and pull your foot up and toward your body. Now, switch by returning the front leg into a downward facing dog position, and complete the same routine for the other side of the body. Upon completion of each side, return legs to the downward dog position. Focus and feel the stretch!

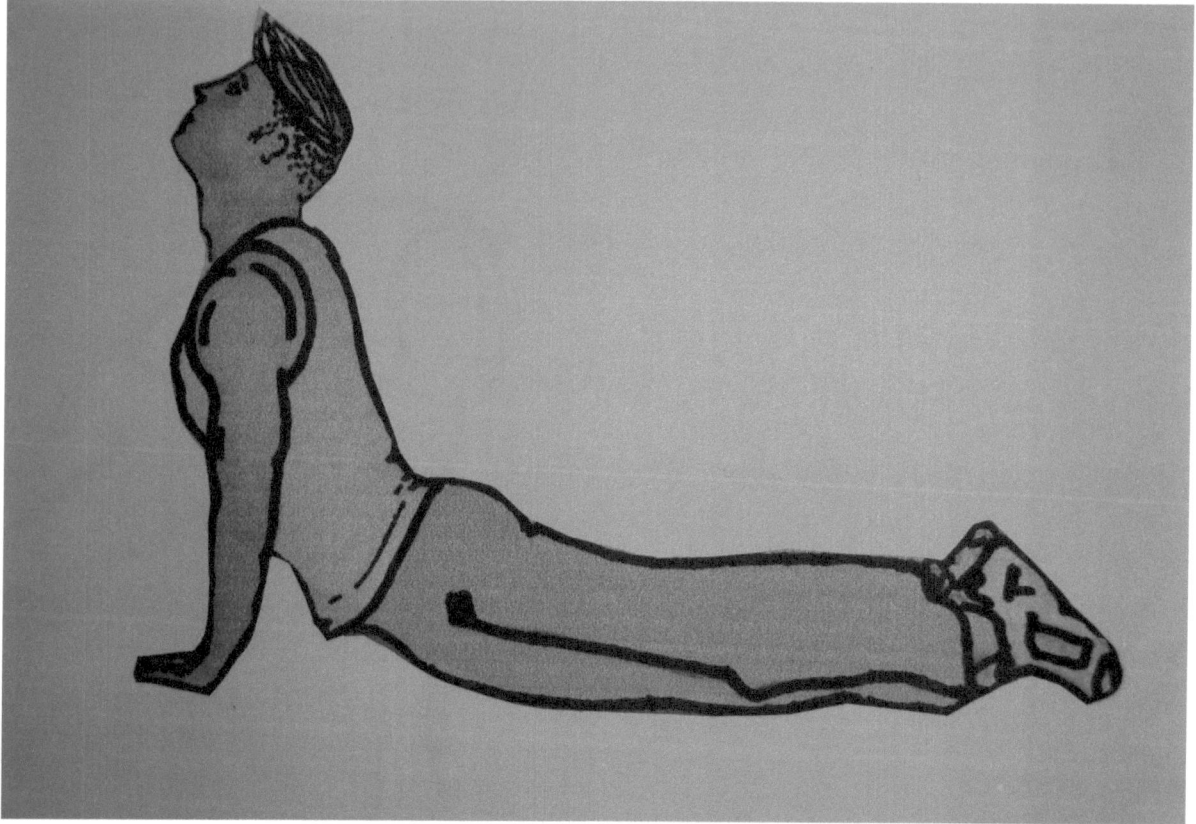

Upward Dog II (2 minutes max) (feet hip distance apart)

Now, move back into an upward dog. Your arms are now supporting your upper torso and you are stretching upward with shoulders down and chest up. You can lean toward each side to feel the stretch in your obliques. You should feel this stretch in both the front and back of your upper body as well as in your legs. Your legs are resting on the mat and your upper body is raised off the floor with the support and strength of your arms. Come out of the downward dog, lean onto one side using one arm to support your body and then roll over to the other side. Focus and feel the stretch!

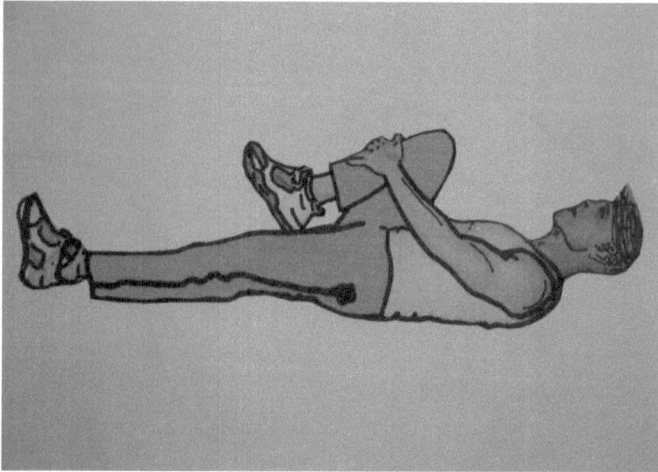
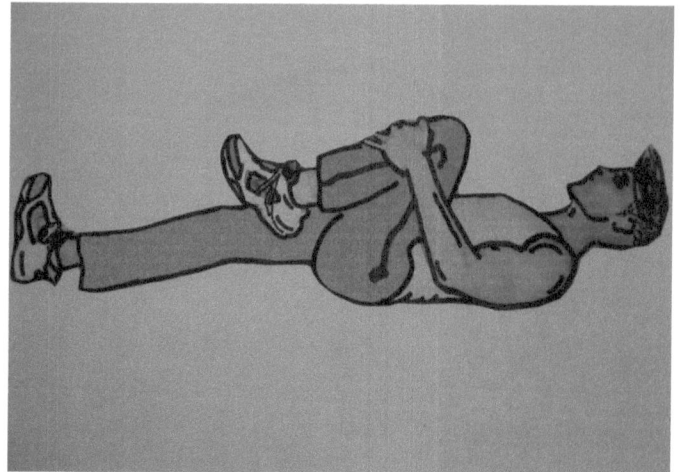
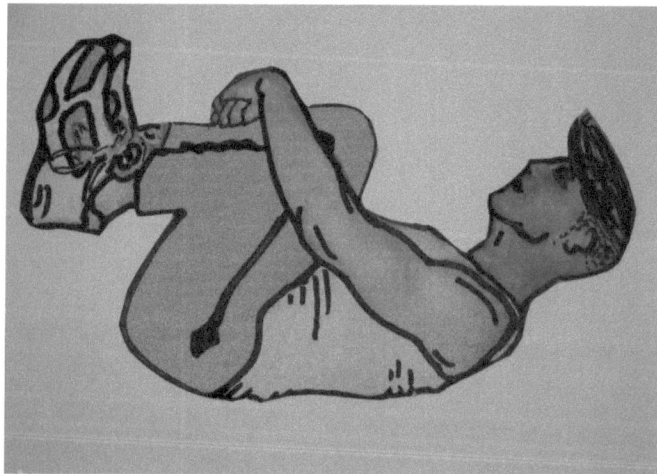

Runner Stretches I (2 minutes max) (feet together)

Lie down on your back and pull one knee up toward your chest and then alternate with the other leg. Next, pull both knees up toward your chest while raising your head toward your knees.

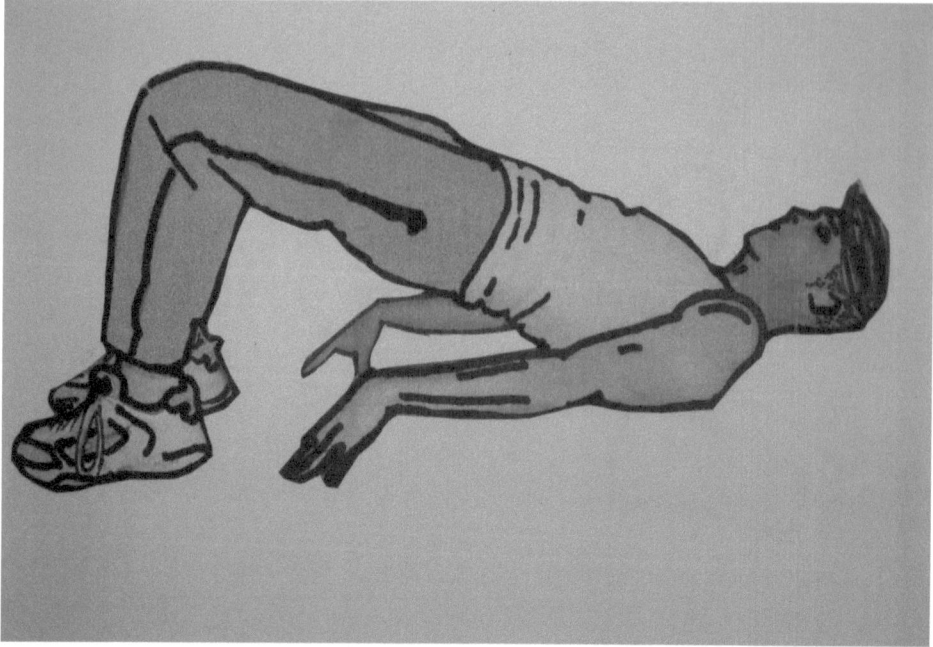

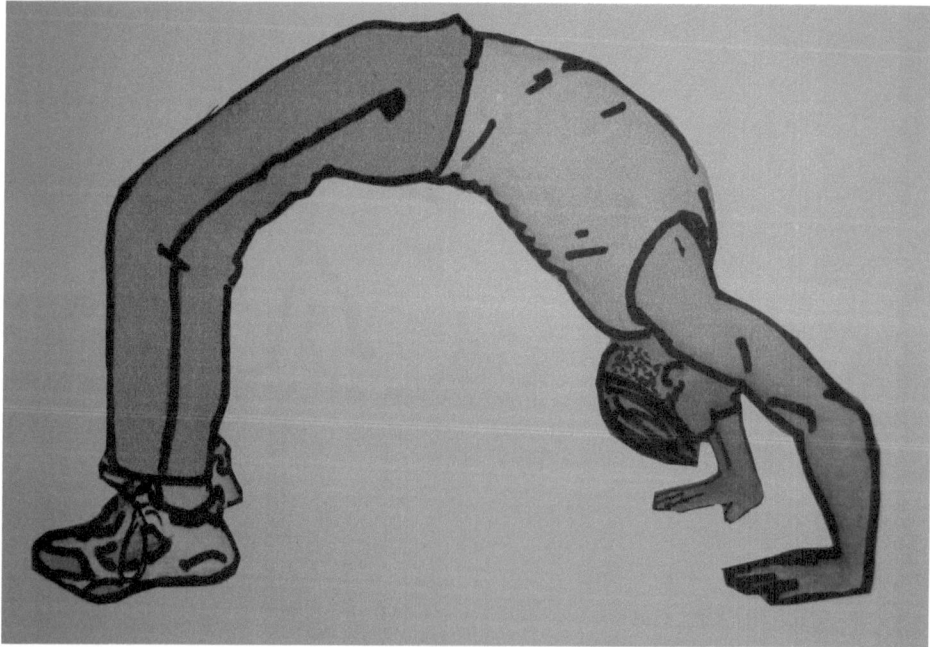

Bridge (2 minutes max) (feet hip distance apart)

Upon coming out of the previous pose, lie down on the mat and raise hips into a modified bridge pose. Upper back is on the ground and hips are pushed upward. This is good for both the lower back and glutes. Then move into a full bridge pose. Hands are placed next to the ears while pushing upwards so that your entire body is off the ground. Focus and feel the stretch!

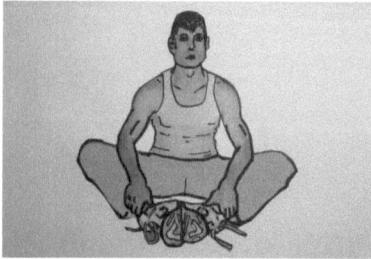
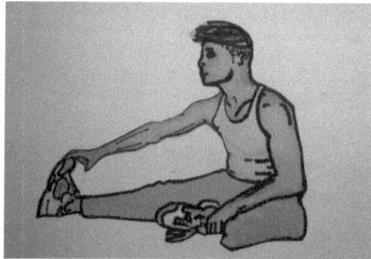
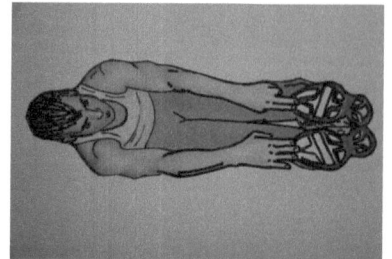
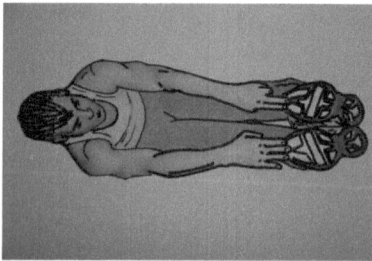
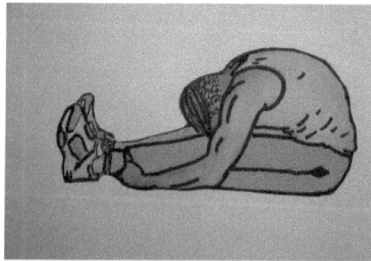
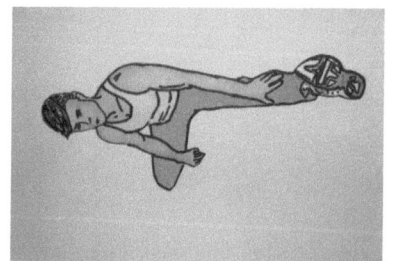
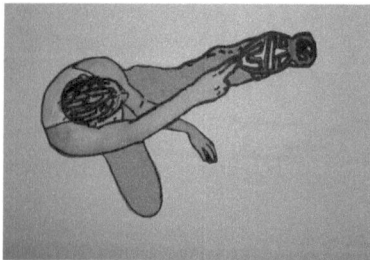
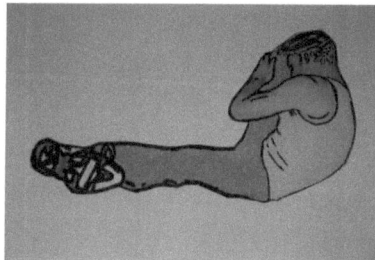
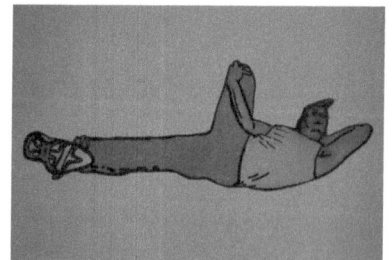

Runner Stretches II (2 minutes max) (feet together)

Now sit up with your knees bent and the soles of your feet pressed together. Lean into knees with your elbows for a thigh stretch. Stretch out one leg with the foot of the other leg pressed into the upper thigh and reach and touch right hand to right foot then switch legs. Then with both legs stretched out in front of you, take a deep breath and release while reaching toward the toes and hold for 10-15 seconds. Focus and feel the stretch!

Now pull one leg back so that you have one outstretched leg and one leg bent almost behind you. Lean your head toward your bent knee. Reach toward your outstretched leg with the opposite arm. Now, place your hand across the back of your neck and lean backwards. Change leg position and repeat. Focus and feel the stretch!

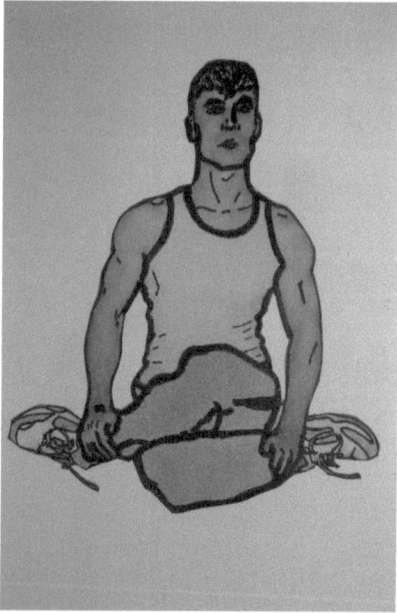
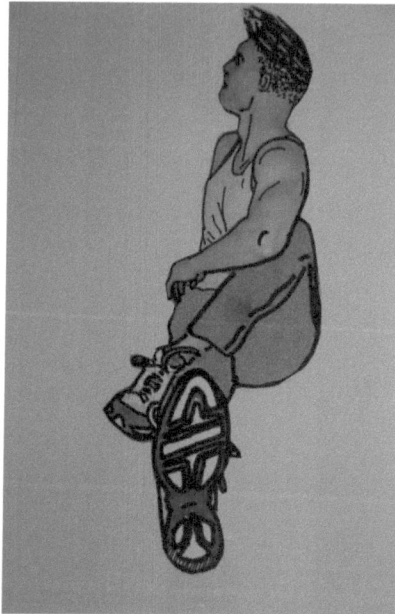
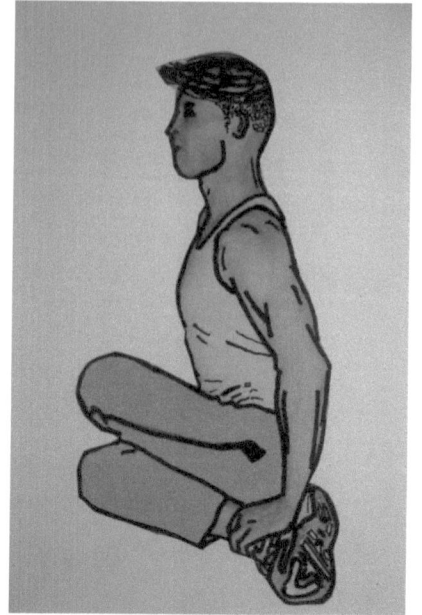
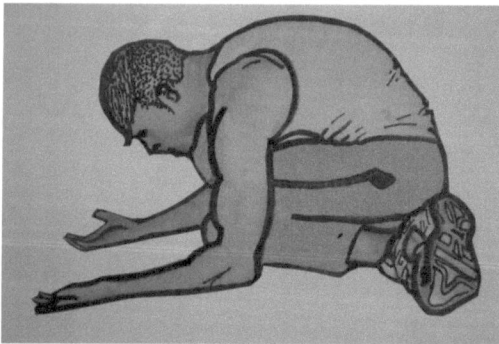
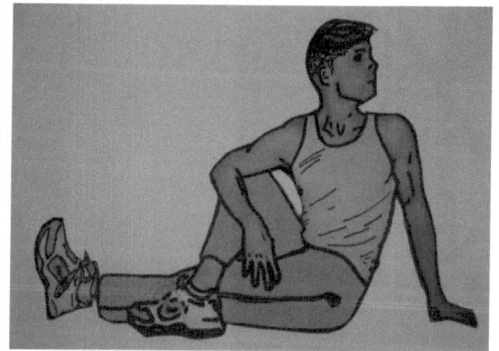

Sit and Twist (2 minutes max)

Now, sit up and cross one leg over the other leg at the knee joint. Stretch your body upward and then lean forward over your knees with your head relaxed. Reverse the leg positions and repeat. Focus and feel the stretch!

Cross one leg over the other so that one knee is on top of the other knee. Sit up straight then lean over your knees so that your chest is leaning on top of your knees with outstretched hands. Switch legs and repeat. Focus and feel the stretch!

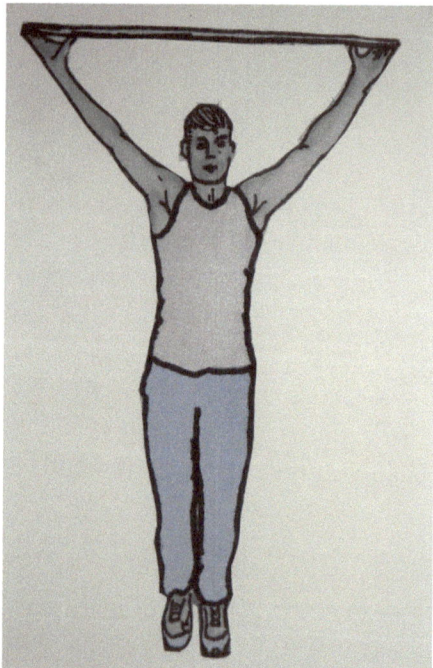
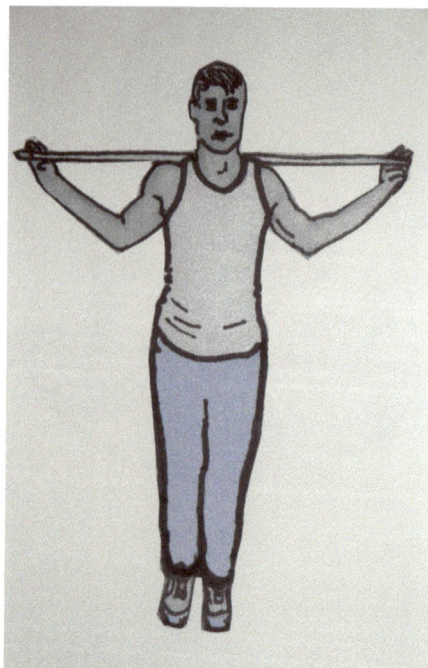
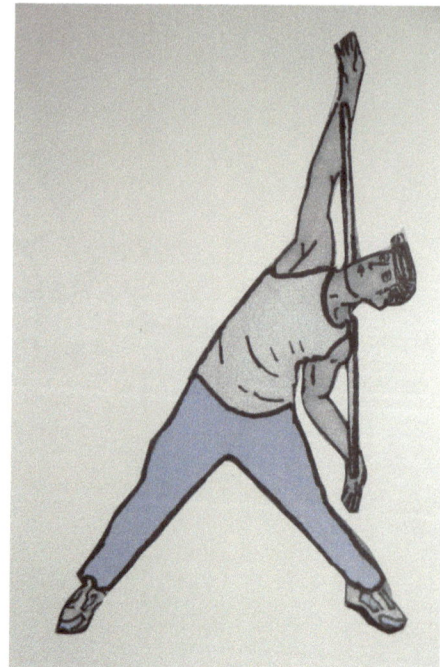
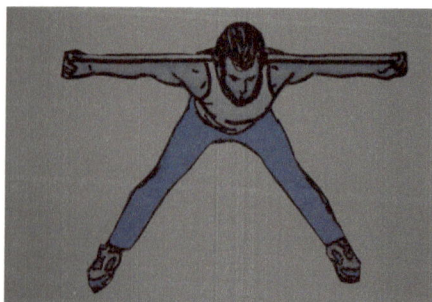
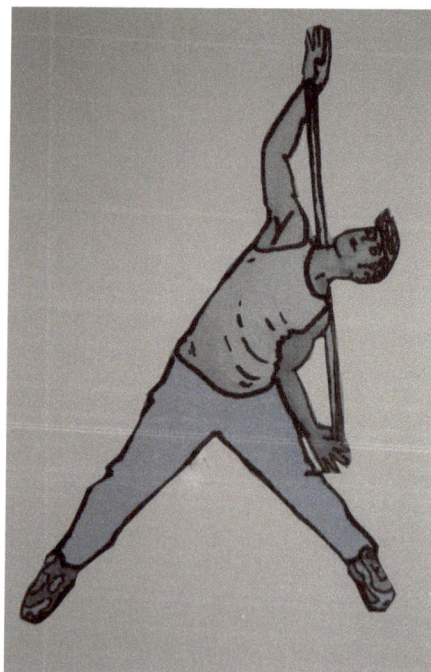
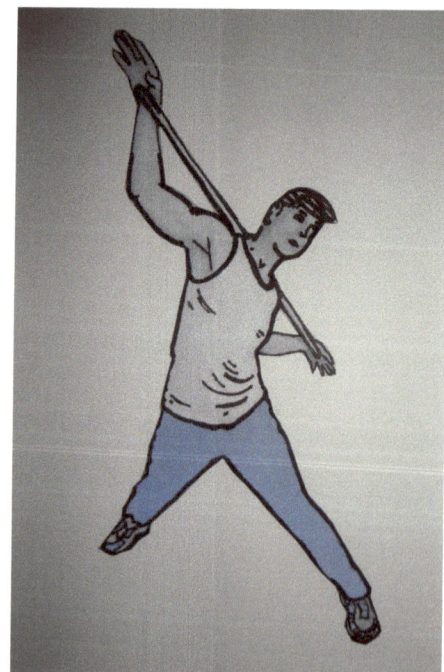

Standing Twists (2 minutes max) (legs hip distant or wider than hip distant apart)

Take a bar and place upon the back of your neck/shoulders. Bend your knees and lean back slightly while twisting with an upper inclination to the twist. Straighten your stance and now lean over from side to side. Next, bend at the waist with knees slightly bent and twist. Finally, stand up again and lean from side to side but with an emphasis upon the bar positioned alternately toward the front and back of the knees. Focus and feel the stretch!

You're finished! Your body and muscles are now warmed up so that you can enjoy your athletic activity of choice safely and free of injury. I also strongly encourage you to engage in a cool down activity when finished with exercising. I have been working out for 27 years and have never experienced any injuries related to working out. I can count on two hands the number of times that I have actually pulled a muscle, and consequently had some soreness but never an injury. I believe that this or any other stretch program is critical to remaining strong, healthy and injury free. I also encourage you to eat well, drink lots of water, and get plenty of sleep. Moderation in everything including sports is key to a balanced lifestyle. Focus and feel the stretch in life!

www.ingramcontent.com/pod-product-compliance
Lightning Source LLC
Chambersburg PA
CBHW060859270326
41935CB00003B/38